PACU Nurse Notes

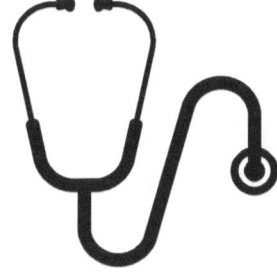

This book belongs to:

_____

coloring Section

I Had Fun Once,Then I Went To Nursing School

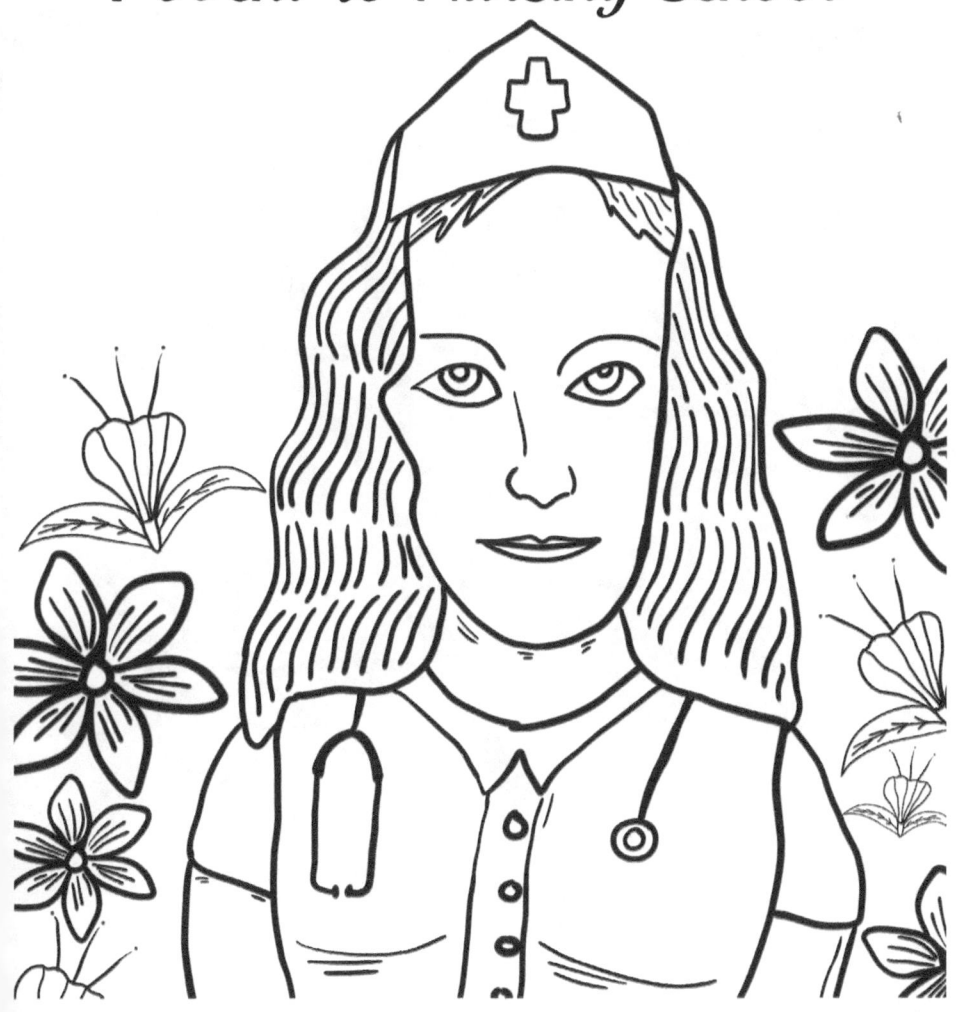

Ativan A Nurse's Best Friend

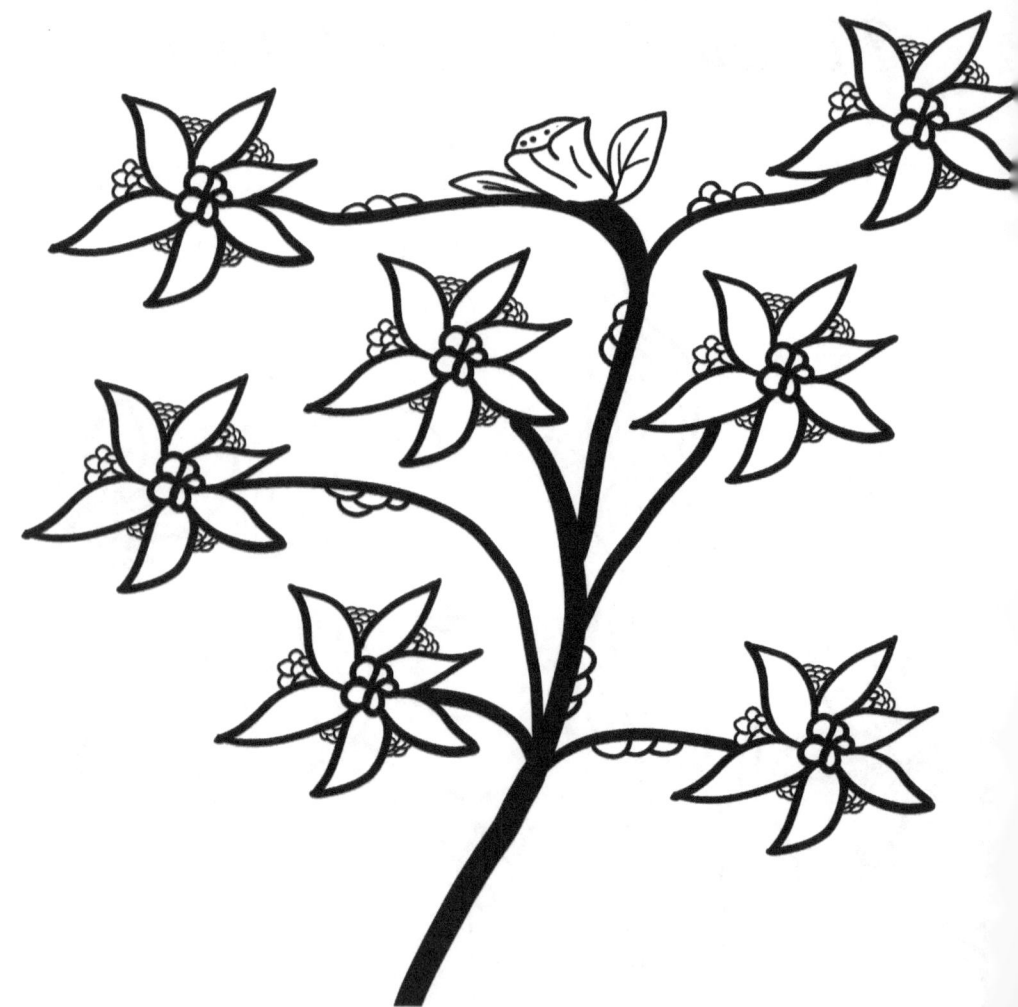

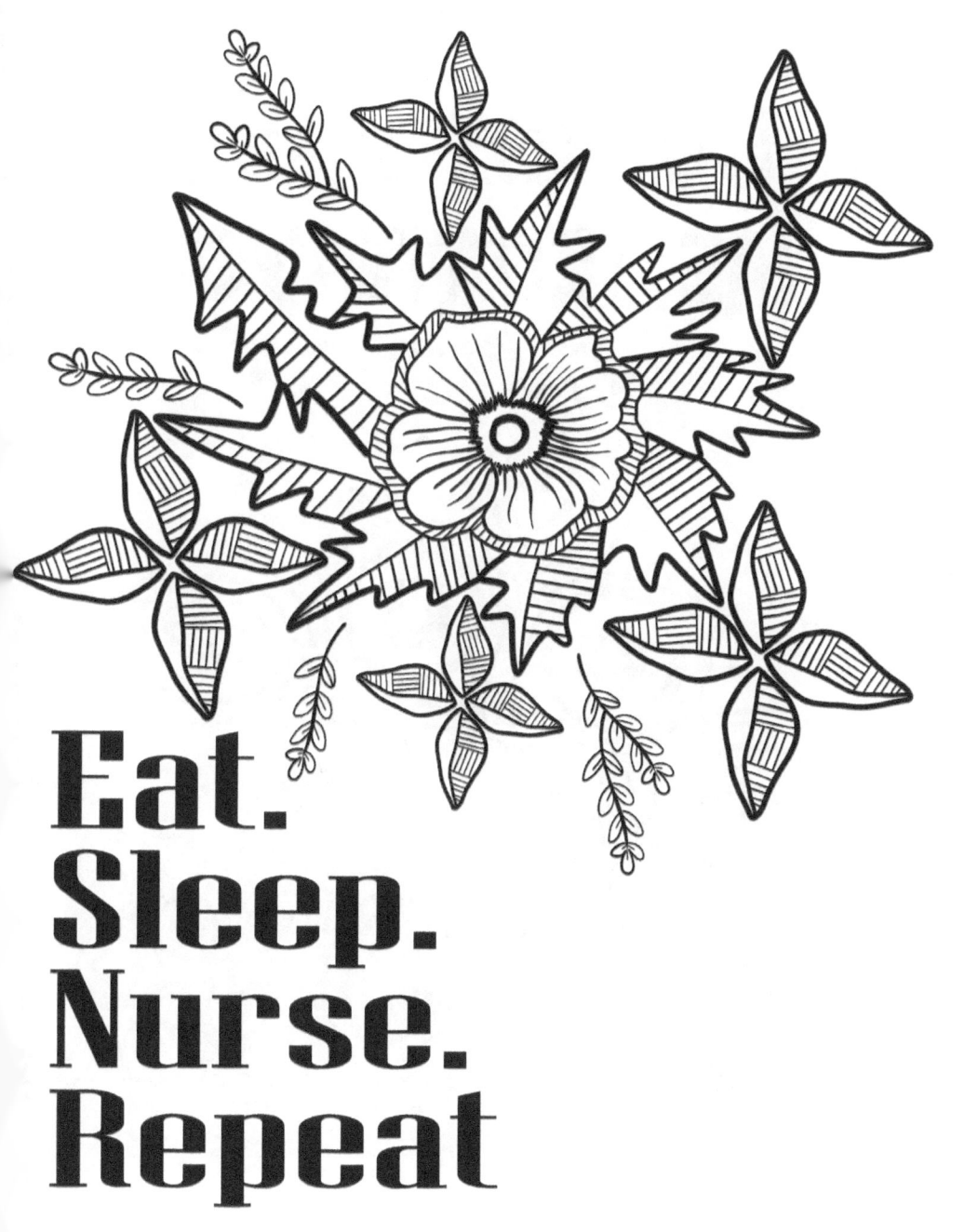

Eat.
Sleep.
Nurse.
Repeat

DO NOT MAKE ME SEDATE YOU.

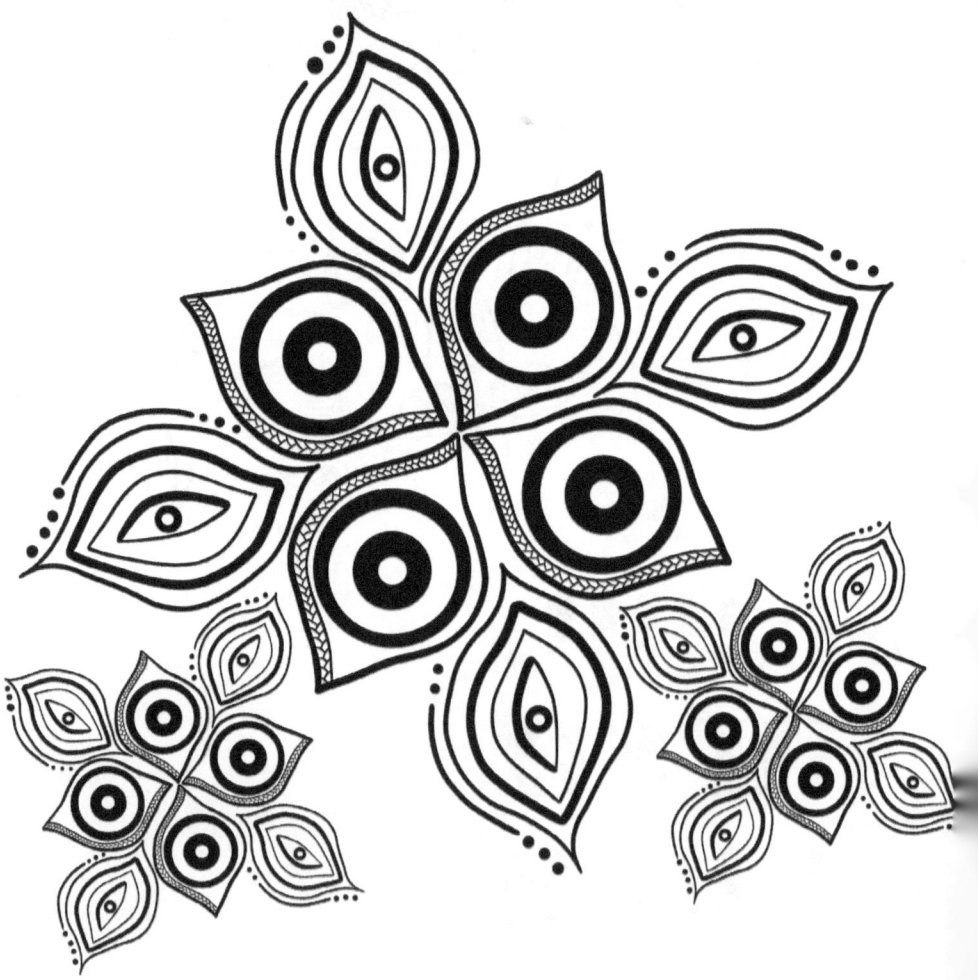

Best Nurse Ever

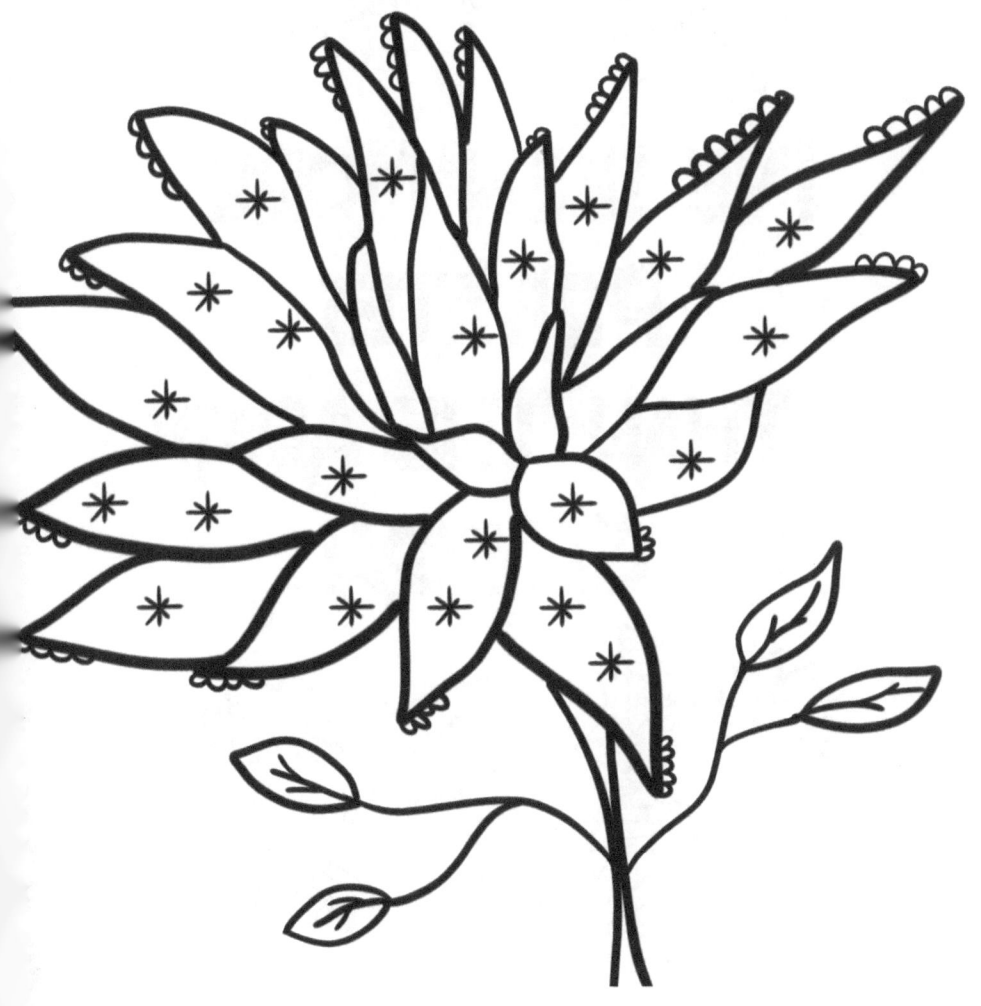

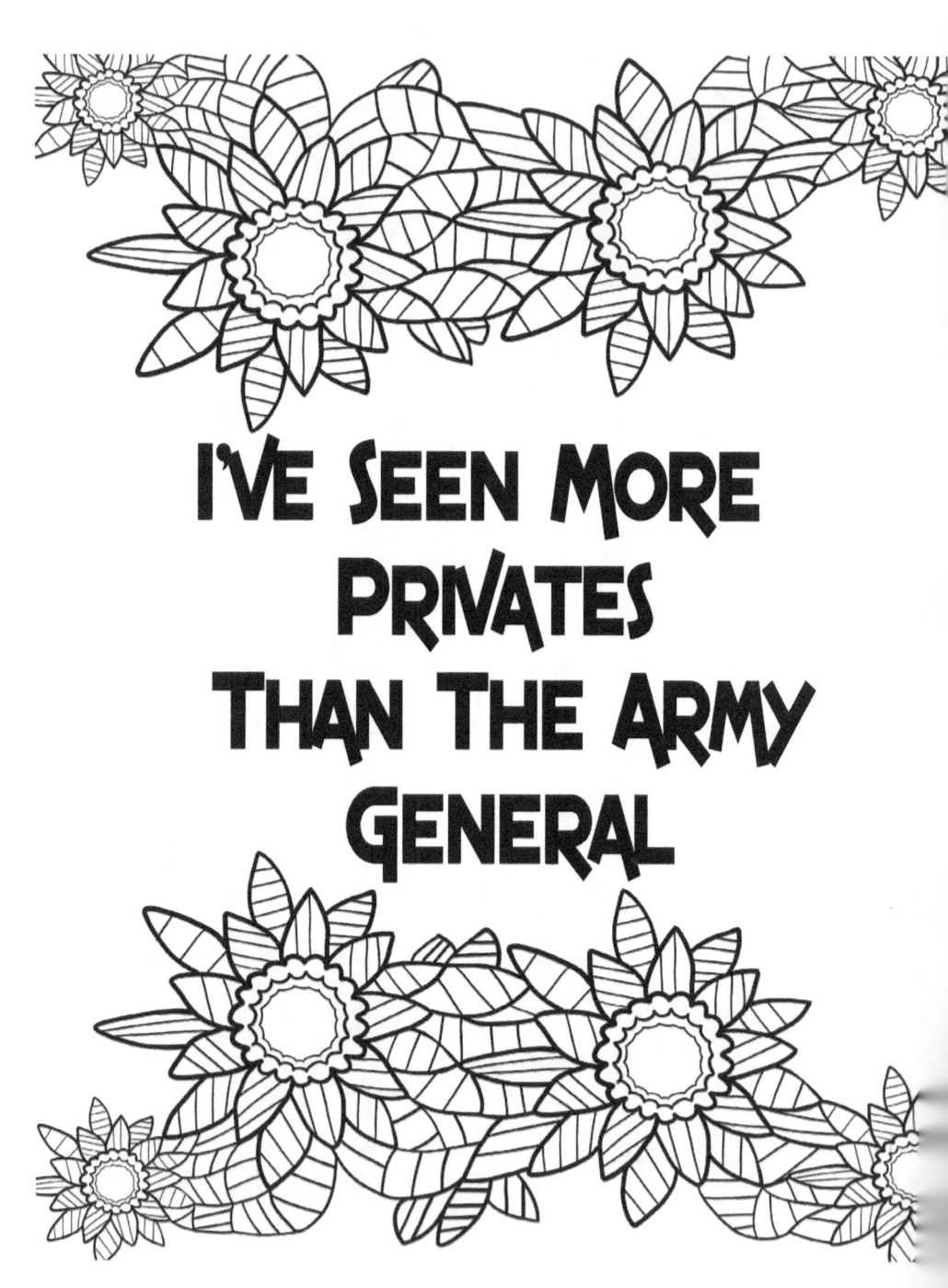

I'VE SEEN MORE PRIVATES THAN THE ARMY GENERAL

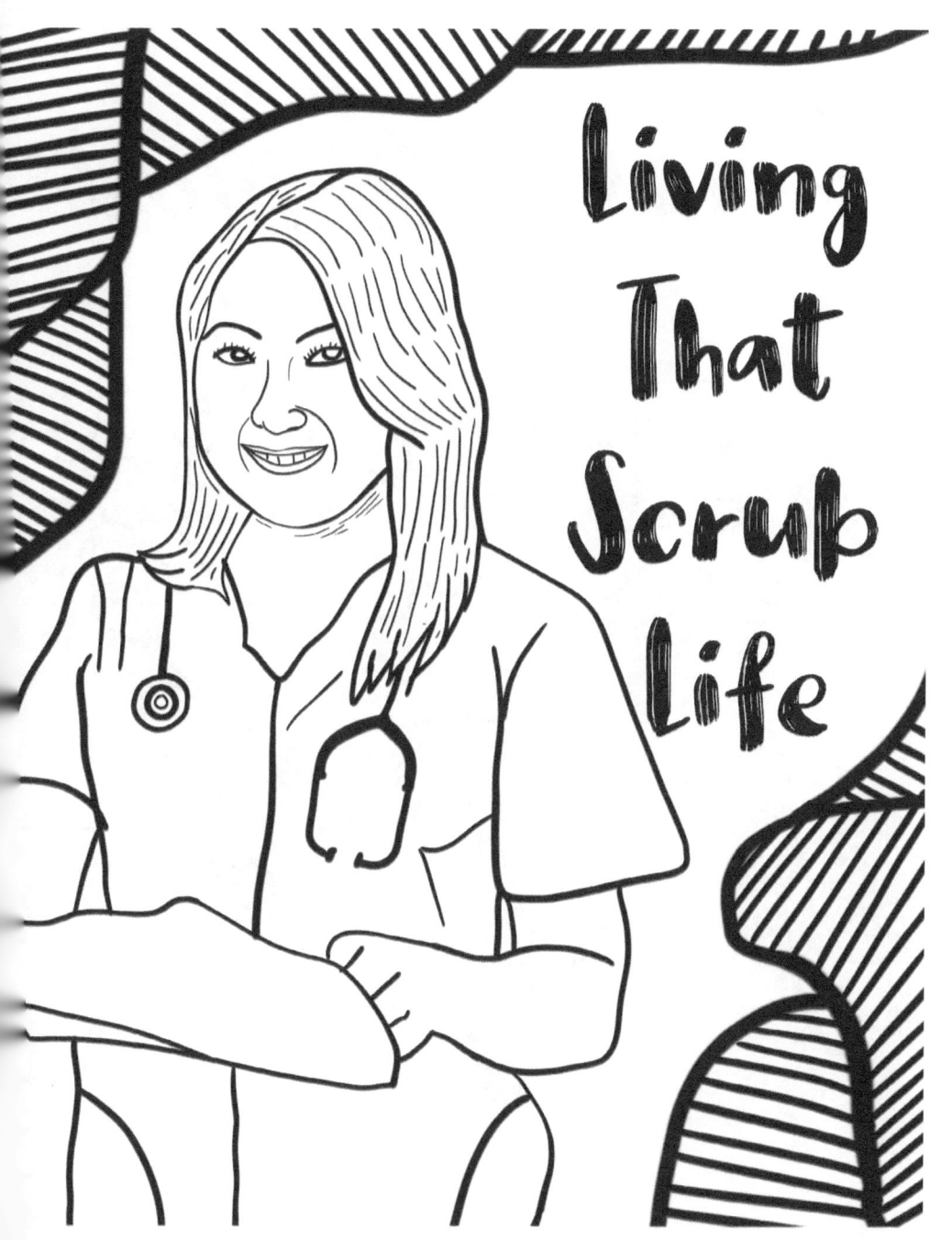

Nurse Squad

If You're Happy and You Know It, It's Your Meds

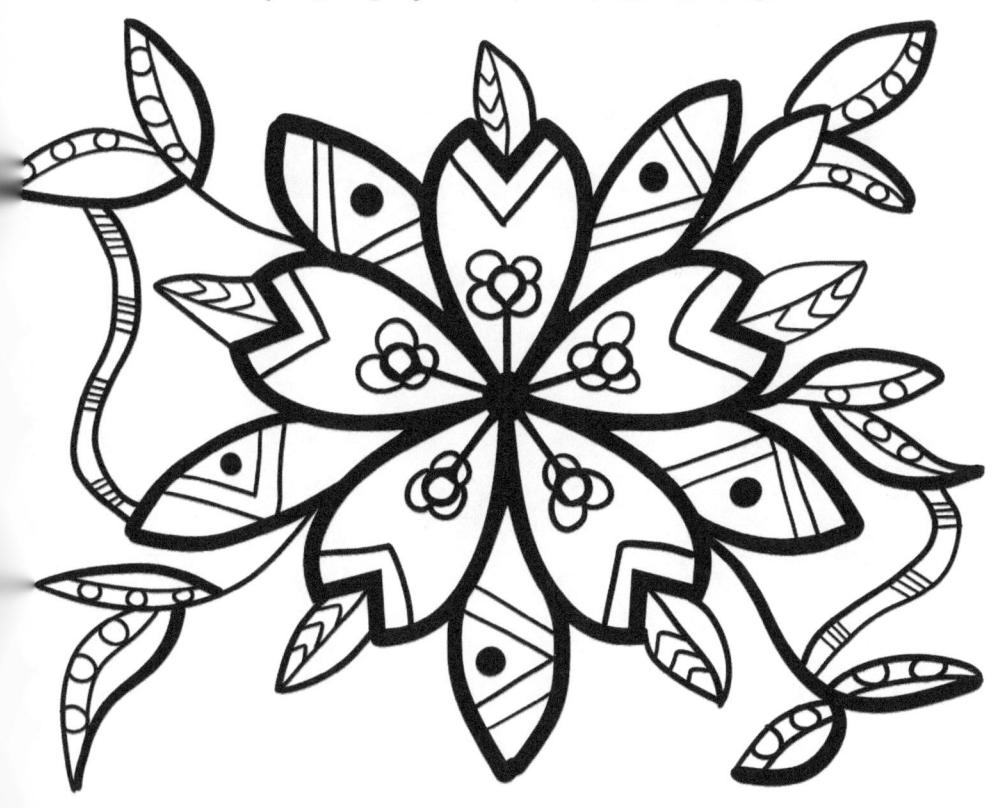